AF294912

SOPHROLOGY FOR BEGINNERS

Simple techniques for relaxation and wellbeing

Written by Vera Smayan
In collaboration with Céline Faidherbe
Translated by Rebecca Neal

Health and Wellbeing 50MINUTES.com

50MINUTES.com

HEALTH AND WELLBEING
WITHOUT THE HEADACHE

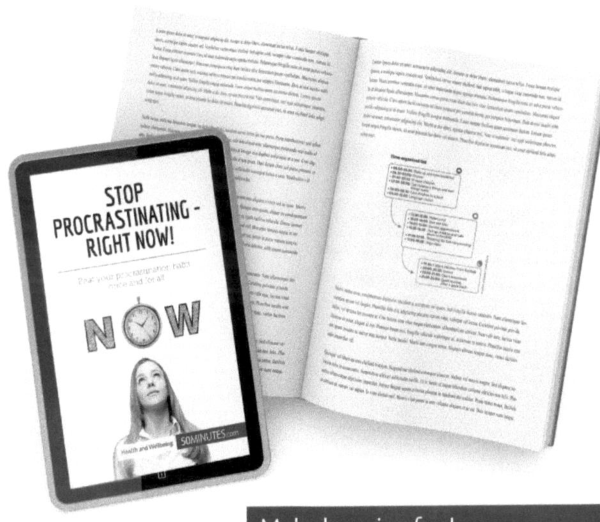

Make learning fun!

Learn to love yourself

Dealing with bullying at school

Your guide to making friends

www.50minutes.com

FURTHER READING 61

SOPHROLOGY FOR BEGINNERS

SIMPLE TECHNIQUES FOR RELAXATION AND WELLBEING

- **Problem:** sophrology aims to restore mental and physical balance through a range of techniques inspired by both Eastern and Western approaches, but the discipline is still relatively little-known. Once you have grasped the basic principles of this method, you will be able to incorporate it into your everyday life for therapeutic purposes and for your personal development.
- **Aims:** to understand the basic principles of sophrology and learn some simple exercises to carry out at home, either to deal with problems such as stress and insomnia or simply to gain a better understanding of your body, relax and boost your overall wellbeing.
- **FAQs:**
  - Is sophrology the same thing as hypnosis?
  - Is sophrology the same thing as meditation,

yoga or psychoanalysis?
- Can I carry out sophrology without the help of a sophrologist?
- Who can carry out sophrology and how does it work?
- How long does a course of sophrology last?
- What happens during a course of sophrology?
- How can I become a Caycedian sophrologist?

Sophrology was developed in the 1960s by the Colombian psychiatrist Alfonso Caycedo (born in 1932) with the help of a team of other doctors and scientists. The term is a neologism which combines three Greek roots: *sos* ("harmony"), *phron* (which is linked to the mind and wisdom) and *logos* ("word", "reason" or "discourse"). The approach synthesises a number of Eastern meditation techniques and Western relaxation methods in order to expand the individual's consciousness and enable them to unlock their full potential.

Sophrology is suitable for individuals of any age and level of fitness, and is equally effective for people who are suffering from illness and people who are in generally good health. It can be used in the treatment of addiction, psychosomatic illnesses and anxiety, and is also helpful as an accompaniment to children's activities and sports.

The main aim of sophrology is to create a sense of harmony between the practitioner's mind and body by reaching a profound state of relaxation on the border between sleep and wakefulness (referred to as the sophroliminal level).

The discipline is based on the principle that our bodies and minds are inextricably linked, and involves physical exercises that aim to strengthen our consciousness and alter our perception of reality. Sophrology raises our awareness of the connections between our body and mind and teaches us that our perception of events is relative and can be changed. This helps us to develop a positive attitude and greater resistance to stress and everyday physical and mental suffering.

Sophrology teaches us to gain a better understanding of ourselves, get back in touch with our feelings, think positively, boost our concentration and manage stress effectively. It also makes us aware of our own potential and can help rebuild our self-confidence, making it an excellent way to maintain inner balance and achieve overall wellbeing.

WHAT IS SOPHROLOGY?

THE HISTORY OF SOPHROLOGY

Sophrology was established in 1960 by the psychiatrist Alfonso Caycedo, an expert in hypnosis, and its popularity has grown steadily ever since. By the 1970s, it was being used in medical and paramedical treatments and being taught in psychiatry faculties in some 60 countries.

Caycedo initially carried out hypnosis alongside some of the psychiatric treatments that were in use at the time (for example, on patients who had undergone electric shock treatment) in hospitals in Spain. However, he soon decided to develop an alternative, more scientifically rigorous method. In 1960, he coined the term "sophrology" and founded the Sophrology Society in Spain.

His meeting with the Swiss psychiatrist Ludwig Binswanger (1881-1966) had a major impact on him as it gave him greater insight into phenomenology, which was developed by the Austrian philosopher Edmund Husserl (1859-

1938). Phenomenology is based on the study of consciousness and aims to break down the division between the mind and body and the feelings and intellect. According to this approach, experience is the best way to grasp the essence of a phenomenon, based on the supposition that phenomena "are what they are" and we can understand their reality through our consciousness.

Caycedo then spent two years travelling in Tibet, India and Japan, where he studied yoga, Zen Buddhism and meditation, which all influence both the body and the mind. The synthesis of physical and mental approaches to consciousness came to form the basis of sophrology. He saw this new discipline as a science and began practising it at the Santa Isabel hospital in Madrid. This marked the beginning of an extensive period of research and experimentation, resulting in Caycedian sophrology®, a holistic treatment approach which allows the individual to attain overall physical and mental balance.

From 1967 onwards, sophrology developed further and increased in effectiveness thanks to the incorporation of other techniques, including:

- autosuggestion, which uses self-induced suggestion to promote positive thinking;
- progressive relaxation, as developed by the American physician Edmund Jacobson (1888-1983), to relax the muscles;
- autogenic training, which was developed by the German psychiatrist Johannes Heinrich Schultz (1884-1970) and uses autosuggestion to promote relaxation.

Sophrology began to attract attention in the medical world after the first international congress on the subject was held in Barcelona in 1970. A few years later, the discipline broadened its scope and began to be used in the social prevention sector. In France, which was one of the first countries to embrace sophrology, training became easier to access, as it was no longer reserved for medical professionals.

Around 20 years later, the Alfonso Caycedo Foundation was established, with its headquarters in Andorra. Sofrocay®, which is headed by Caycedo's daughter Natalia Caycedo, who is also a psychiatrist, oversees all the sophrology schools in Europe to ensure their quality (in total, there are some 50 schools located in Belgium, Spain, France, Italy, Portugal and Switzerland).

From this point onwards, the discipline began to diversify. While Caycedian sophrology® continued to take a philosophical, spiritual approach, other branches which focused more on social and therapeutic uses began to develop in France. These approaches differ from Caycedian sophrology® in that they incorporate other techniques, including cognitivism, neuro-linguistic programming (NLP), massage and yoga.

Nowadays, there are practitioners and schools of sophrology all over the world and the discipline is recognised by numerous psychiatry faculties, but it is still not officially regulated. Nonetheless, there is a sophrologists' trade union which ensures that all members hold valid professional qualifications.

A DISCIPLINE TO STRENGTHEN CONSCIOUSNESS

The initial motto of the sophrology movement was *Ut conscientia noscatur* (Latin for "So that consciousness is known"), which perfectly encapsulates its aims. It uses mental and physical techniques to study human consciousness and its potential, and serves numerous purposes: prevention, treatment, therapy, pedagogical intervention and rehabilitation in the fields of mental health and psychosomatic illnesses. It is employed in both clinical and social settings.

Caycedo defines consciousness as a kind of transcendent life energy which combines mental and physical elements in a unified whole.

Sophrology and Plato's Allegory of the Cave

In his dialogue *The Republic*, Plato (Greek philosopher, 5th century BCE) uses the famous Allegory of the Cave to represent humanity's ignorance. Caycedo drew inspiration from it to define sophrology and the role of each participant in the method.

In Plato's allegory, a group of people have lived chained together facing the wall of a gloomy cave for their entire lives. All they can see are shadows, which they take to be reality. One day, one of them is taken outside into the light, and although they are initially blinded by it, they are eventually able to see the outside world and do not want to return to their former condition of slavery. If they were to return to the cave to free the other people there, they would not be able to see anything because their eyes have adjusted to the light. Moreover, their companions would probably not believe them: instead, they would think that they had gone mad and turn against them. Having spent their entire lives in darkness, they would find it impossible to believe that everything they had ever seen was no more than an illusion and true reality was outside the cave.

According to Caycedo, sophrology allows individuals to free themselves from their chains and step outside the cave by developing their consciousness so that they can distinguish between illusions and reality. The individual is a truth-seeker, while the sophrologist serves as their guide in their journey of liberation and self-discovery.

Heightened self-awareness

Regularly practising sophrology increases the individual's awareness of their own body, mind, emotional states and personal values. This self-discovery, which is accomplished through simple relaxation and visualisation exercises, fosters optimism, enthusiasm for life and the development of positive attitudes towards oneself and others. Some sophrology techniques promote vitality and energy, while others assist with relaxation. Regular practice enables users to develop their attention span, concentration and memory, and to attain mental and physical balance.

WHAT FIELDS IS SOPHROLOGY USED IN?

Sophrology is employed in the medical, para-medical (clinical sophrology) and social (preventative sophrology) fields. Within each of these fields, the method is used in a range of areas:

- **Medical settings:** in the treatment of physical and mental illnesses, preparation for childbirth, preparation for surgery and physiotherapy.
- **Educational settings:** to boost self-esteem, concentration and memory, and to defuse situations involving aggression and violence.
- **The sports sector:** to boost performance, concentration and motivation, control fear, improve blood circulation and recover quicker from muscle fatigue.

- **Personal issues:** in the management of relationship problems, conflict management, treatment of addiction and stress, the promotion of self-confidence and personal fulfilment.
- **Professional settings:** in personnel and stress management, and to increase motivation at work and boost concentration and lucidity.

Sophrology can be carried out for individuals and groups, and both adults and teenagers can benefit from it. Its most frequent applications include:

- anger and emotional management;
- stress management;
- the treatment of eating disorders;
- the treatment of sleep problems;
- improvement of general quality of life.

THE BASIC PRINCIPLES OF SOPHROLOGY

PROGRESSIVE METHODOLOGY

Sophrology is based on Eastern relaxation techniques, and places particular emphasis on the "active principle" (for example, attention to points of contact on the body) in order to strengthen its effects. This has resulted in the development of a series of basic exercises, which are used to restore physical and mental balance, as well as around 100 specific exercises, which are based on self-observation and aim to treat a host of problems, ranging from problems linked to stress to increasing lung function and blood circulation.

The techniques of sophrology can be divided into two categories: dynamic techniques (physical exercises) and static techniques (visualisation and meditation). Dynamic techniques include sophronisation (physical and mental relaxation) and the 12 degrees of dynamic relaxation, which are further divided into numerous sub-degrees.

Sophrology is based on a progressive approach, and the dynamic relaxation exercises and specific techniques enable practitioners to go through three steps at their own pace:

- discovery;
- conquest;
- transformation.

In practice, sophrology involves combining dynamic relaxation exercises and specific techniques based on the individual's personal circumstances. Each session follows a set order: sophronisation, dynamic relaxation exercises/ specific techniques, desophronisation.

The sophrologist will establish a program based on their patient's needs and objectives. This will involve discovery techniques for the first few sessions, before moving on to conquest and transformation exercises.

DYNAMIC RELAXATION

Dynamic relaxation is structured as a series of exercises which are subdivided into degrees. In Caycedian sophrology®, there are 12 degrees in total, the first four of which are common to all branches of sophrology:

- the first degree improves concentration and awareness of the body;
- the second degree increases physical self-awareness;
- the third degree incorporates meditation and is always carried out in the presence of a sophrologist;
- the fourth degree develops the person's individual and existential values, and is generally carried out as part of a group.

In Caycedian sophrology®, dynamic relaxation is divided into three cycles:

- the reduction cycle (the first, second, third and fourth degrees of dynamic relaxation); this is the phase of concentration during which the sophrologist teaches the patient to become aware of the muscle contractions that occur during movement;
- the radical cycle (the fifth, sixth, seventh and eighth degrees of dynamic relaxation); this is the contemplative phase, which is based on the contemplation of the body;

- the existential cycle (the ninth, tenth, eleventh and twelfth degrees of dynamic relaxation); this is the meditation phase, which is inspired by Zen Buddhism but does not have a religious or spiritual dimension.

The repetition of the same relaxation techniques allows the practitioner to progress from one phase to the next.

LIFE-ENHANCING EXPERIENCES

Life-enhancing experiences (referred to in French by the neologism "vivance") are experiences in which naturally occurring phenomena are absorbed into the individual's consciousness. Didier-Patrick Beudaert explains that "vivance" exemplifies the difference between existing and living, and uses the example of going to a restaurant with a very good friend and creating great memories that will stay with you for a long time.

The techniques of sophrology encourage life-enhancing experiences, and by repeating these kinds of experiences, we undergo a period of transformation and move closer to a state of balance between our body and mind.

THE BODY MAP AS LIVED REALITY

In sophrology, the idea of the body map includes the image of the body (meaning the objective representation of the body in time and space) and the subjective representation of it (meaning a self-image that is linked to affective and emotional factors, history and socio-cultural elements). As such, the body map can be described as an awareness of our bodies, but also as a lived reality, which is fundamental to human experience as everything (feelings, emotions, etc.) is connected to the body.

If these two representations of the body are unbalanced, our body map is disturbed. Awareness techniques which direct the practitioner's attention to their senses with the aim of enabling them to fully focus on their body constitute the first degree of dynamic relaxation.

Sophrology enables practitioners to gain a greater awareness of their bodies, accept their uniqueness and engage positively with the world around them, which in turn benefits their relationships.

POSITIVE ACTION

According to sophrology, any positive action which affects our minds also has an effect on our bodies, and vice versa. In this case, "positive" means any action which increases vitality and awareness or has a beneficial effect on our health, including feelings and emotions inspired by everyday events (which can be as simple as our morning coffee or memories of the past).

The techniques of sophrology aim to strengthen positive, vital elements in order to increase the individual's overall fulfilment.

THE SOPHROLIMINAL LEVEL

Caycedo uses the term "sophroliminal level" to refer to the state between sleep and wakefulness, when our brain is calm and receptive and we experience things with a relaxed but alert state of mind. This state is conducive to the conditioning of our consciousness, as our imagination and concentration are very active. It is a sensitive time that we can use to strengthen the positive aspects of our lives.

All sophrology sessions begin with basic sophronisation exercises to enable the practitioner to
enter the sophroliminal level.

THE *TERPNOS LOGOS*

Terpnos logos is an ancient Greek expression
which literally means "soft speaking", and it ap-
pears as early as Plato's dialogue the *Charmides*
(c. 388 BCE). It is linked to *thumos* (a Greek word
expressing the concept of "spiritedness") and
allows the individual to enter a state of profound
mental calm and concentration.

In sophrology, *terpnos logos* refers to the way the
sophrologist speaks: slowly, in a neutral tone,
at a constant volume and in a way that is both
repetitive and personalised (through specific
vocabulary which serves to preserve the practitioner's individuality). They also pause at the
end of each exercise, which allows the individual
to absorb the experience they have just gone
through. *Terpnos logos* is a fundamental tool
for the sophrologist as they guide their patient
through the exercises of sophrology.

HOW TO PRACTISE SOPHROLOGY

When you practise sophrology, you will carry out part of the work under the supervision of a trained sophrologist and do some independent personal development work each day. The sophrologist will tell you which exercises to do based on your objectives, and they will change each week.

To carry out these exercises, you need to be able to isolate yourself for 10 to 20 minutes in a calm environment where you will not be interrupted by any distractions (telephone, open windows, etc.).

When you work with the sophrologist, they will guide you through exercises which will enable you to change your behaviour based on your desired goal.

The relationship between the sophrologist and their patient is collaborative. There is no physical contact between them and the patient will not be forced to do anything. The treatment progressively evolves and is tailored to the individual, with the sophrologist serving as their guide as they work towards a higher level of consciousness.

Before beginning the series of exercises, the sophrologist will carry out a preliminary interview in which they will ask their patient questions in order to obtain an overview of their physical and mental health, as well as to gain insight into aspects of their life such as their personal history, family environment and day-to-day activities. Sometimes, this is carried out via a detailed questionnaire, which has the advantage of enabling people who struggle to express themselves to give precise answers.

Next, the patient gets into a comfortable position and follows the instructions that the sophrologist gives them in a slow, soft voice (*terpnos logos*). In general, a sophrology session begins with basic sophronisation, then progresses to dynamic relaxation and/or specific techniques, before finishing with desophronisation.

At the end of each session, the sophrologist gives the patient recordings (which are generally sent by email) and diagrams to help them with the exercises they will carry out at home.

There are different approaches to the protocol regarding sophrology sessions. For example, music and decoration are not permitted in Caycedian sophrology® but form an integral part of the treatment in other branches of sophrology.

There are also a number of books and websites that enable users to carry out sophrology sessions independently. However, although some exercises (notably the first degree dynamic relaxation exercises and some specific exercises) can easily be carried out from the comfort of your home, a complete course of sophrology requires the guidance of a specialist.

OVER TO YOU

In a course of sophrology, it is always recommended to keep a journal where you keep track of your training for the week, noting any impressions, feelings and reflections that you had during the sessions, as well as comments about any potential consequences during your sleeping and waking hours. Below is an example of the kind of table you could use in your journal.

	1	2	3	4	5	6	7
Day							
Time							
Exercise							
Positive impressions							
Negative impressions							
Comments (awake)							
Comments (asleep)							

© 50MINUTES.com

ABDOMINAL BREATHING

Abdominal breathing is a preliminary exercise to prepare for any sophrology session, as well as an effective way to relax that can be carried out anywhere and at any time. Babies naturally breathe like this, as do adults while they are sleeping. It is very calming and relaxes the diaphragm.

During the day, find a place where you can be undisturbed for a few minutes and get into a comfortable position, whether this means sitting, lying down or standing up. Start by breathing in through your nose and letting your stomach expand, then breathing out through your nose and letting your stomach go down, taking deep breaths and maintaining a slow rhythm throughout. You will need to practise progressively each day for at least a week. Start by aiming for a few minutes of sustained abdominal breathing, and over time it will become easier and you will be able to keep going for longer.

You will gradually be able to observe the benefits of abdominal breathing not only while you are awake, but also during sleep.

BASIC SOPHRONISATION AND DESOPHRONISATION

Sophronisation is the introductory phase of any sophrology session. It involves visualisation exercises which are guided by the sophrologist's voice and serve to gradually relax the body. Through physical and mental relaxation, the patient can reach the sophroliminal level. This exercise accompanies each dynamic relaxation exercise and specific technique. The exercise concludes with desophronisation, which restores muscle tone and alertness through deep breathing exercises, eye movements and stretching.

<u>PRACTISING BASIC SOPHRONISATION AT HOME</u>

To carry out a shortened version of basic sophronisation (five minutes) at home, you will need to record the *terpnos logos* in advance. The first step is to prepare your text, which you should read slowly in a gentle, monotonous voice, leaving a pause after you mention each part of the body. You can personalise the example below to suit your needs:

> *"We're getting comfortable and closing our eyes... Let's take the time to centre ourselves... We can relax every part of our body through our breathing... We're relaxing our head first... Then our face... (etc.) We are becoming aware of this part of our body... Next we're relaxing the muscles in our neck... in our shoulders... in our arms... (etc.) We are*

The aim is to relax each part of your body, beginning with your head (scalp, forehead and temples, eyebrows, nose, eyelids, eyes, cheeks, jaw, lips, inside of the mouth, tongue) before descending to your back (shoulder blades, spinal column, dorsal and lumbar region, thorax, waist), hips, thighs, knees, lower legs and finally feet.

During the exercise, relax your breathing and focus on the different feelings you experience, making sure that you maintain a curious, open attitude.

At the end of the exercise, you will need to include a desophronisation section, for example:

You are now ready to carry out the exercise. Get into a comfortable position, do a few minutes of abdominal breathing and follow the instructions on your recording.

This shortened form of basic sophronisation is a simple, effective relaxation technique that can help you to increase your overall balance.

SOME BASIC SOPHRONISATION EXERCISES

Reoxygenation exercise

Take a deep breath in, letting your stomach fill with air, and raise your shoulders. Hold the air in for a few seconds, then breathe out and relax your shoulders. Repeat at least three times, relaxing a little more each time. Next, sit down and observe the sensation of the blood beginning to flow again in your legs.

An exercise to increase your spatial awareness

Sit up with your back straight, then begin abdominal breathing and carry out basic sophronisation. Once you have reached the sophroliminal level, take a deep breath, letting your stomach fill with air, and slowly raise your arms to shoulder height. Hold your breath and keep your arms up for a few seconds while visualising your position. Next, breathe out through your mouth to empty your lungs and slowly lower your arms. Try to visualise your movement.

Repeat three times, observing the difference between tension and relaxation, the sensations you feel and your perception of the space around you, which should change over time. Take a small break, then carry out desophronisation.

SPECIFIC TECHNIQUES

These techniques complement the relaxation techniques and have specific goals, such as strengthening or diminishing a particular emotion. They can be subdivided into four main categories:

- Techniques for the present, which deal with issues such as our ability to relax and the management of unpleasant emotions (see Exercise to strengthen a quality, Exercise to displace negative elements and Exercises to improve sleep).

- Techniques for the past, which use positive images or situations from the past to increase our awareness of and control over phenomena (see Exercise to encourage positive elements and Exercise to boost vitality).
- Techniques for the future, which enable us to prepare for a future event (see Exercise to visualise the future and Exercises to reduce stress).
- Integration techniques, which aim to incorporate the past, present and future into a unified whole. These techniques are not for beginners, as they are quite complex.

Exercise to strengthen a quality

This exercise should be carried out twice per day during the daytime. Make sure you are sitting comfortably with your back straight and begin with abdominal breathing before moving on to basic sophronisation. Once you have reached the sophroliminal level, focus on a quality that you want to strengthen and say it in your head every time you breathe out. When you are satisfied with the exercise, move on to desophronisation by gradually moving your muscles and breathing deeply.

Exercise to displace negative elements

This is a simple exercise which can be carried out automatically on a daily basis to manage stress or lessen the intensity of an emotion. It aims to displace any negative elements, meaning anything which is damaging to our lives and which manifests in physical tension and intrusive thoughts.

This exercise removes anything negative from the body. After carrying out basic sophronisation in either a seated or a standing position, breathe in and hold air in your lungs while gently contracting the muscles in your upper body and observing any tension or pain. When you breathe out, completely relax your muscles and let the tension leave your body.

When you go back to breathing normally, imagine that all the negativity is leaving your body. To help with this, you can visualise an image, such as smoke or a dark cloud drifting away from you. Repeat three times, paying close attention to how you feel.

Exercises to improve sleep

Sleep problems are a sign that our mental and physical balance has been disturbed. They are often caused by unhealthy habits during our waking hours, such as a poor diet, a lack of physical activity and too much stress. Breathing well is the first step towards sleeping well. Conscious breathing floods our body with oxygen, which facilitates the elimination of toxins, helps our muscles to relax and strengthens our immune system.

Practising abdominal breathing several times a day is a good way of preparing to go to bed completely relaxed. You can take small breaks of a minute at a time throughout the day to carry out the reoxygenation exercise.

If you still have intrusive thoughts that are stopping you from sleeping, try the following exercises:

• While you are lying down in bed, carry out abdominal breathing and basic sophronisation. Once you have reached the sophroliminal level, pay attention to your body position, your body's points of contact with the mattress and the feeling of the sheets on your skin. Next, carry out the exercise to displace negative elements: imagine that each time you breathe out, you are expelling some tension and that all your worries and negative thoughts are leaving your body like a cloud or a puff of smoke. Repeat three times.

- Breathe in for a count of three and out for a count of four, then breathe lightly with your lungs empty for a count of three and begin the cycle again. Repeat the exercise at your own pace until you feel a sense of calm. Next, begin the exercise to encourage positive elements: imagine that you are in a place you like, where you feel happy and at peace. Use all five of your senses and take time to really immerse yourself in this place. Embrace the sense of peace that this brings and imagine that calm is spreading through your body every time you breathe out.

Exercise to encourage positive elements

This is an energising exercise that enables us to activate the presence of positive elements in our bodies. By this we mean anything that boosts our wellbeing, such as emotions, feelings and memories. This exercise allows us to recognise anything that brings positivity into our lives and boost its effects, resulting in increased self-confidence, a state of general wellbeing and a positive attitude towards everyday life.

Begin by sitting with your back straight and carrying out basic sophronisation. Then, breathe in and hold the air in your lungs while gently contracting the muscles in your upper body and observing any places where you feel tension or pain. When you breathe out, relax your muscles and let the tension leave your body.

Once you have done this, think about an image, situation or word that you associate with positivity. Now that you have chosen your positive thought, link it to your breathing: embrace it as you breathe in and let it spread through your upper body as you breathe out. Repeat at least five times, paying close attention to the exercise's beneficial effects. Next, focus on the feeling of wellbeing that is spreading through your body. Finish with desophronisation to return to a more alert state.

Exercise to boost vitality

This is a classic energising exercise to carry out during the day, ideally in the morning after having breakfast.

After carrying out abdominal breathing and using basic sophronisation to reach the sophroliminal level, go through the exercise to encourage positive elements. Close your eyes and imagine that you are somewhere sunny. Imagine that each time you breathe in you are also breathing in rays of sunlight and the energy of the sun, and that each time you breathe out this energy is spreading throughout your body, warming and energising you as it flows through your head, shoulders, arms, legs and feet. Visualise this for several minutes before moving on to desophronisation.

Exercise to visualise the future

This is a way of developing attributes that you will need in the future and of preparing to face a specific moment (such as an exam or childbirth). The exercise outlined below will allow you to visualise a future event, and can be carried out without the assistance of a sophrologist.

Sit down with your back straight and carry out basic sophronisation. Once you have reached the sophroliminal level, carry out the exercise to displace negative elements. You are now ready to visualise the future. You will need a pre-recorded *terpnos logos* as follows:

> "Now, we can focus on the future situation we want to prepare for... We are imagining ourselves experiencing this situation, without focusing on the details, but following its progression as though we were watching a film... We are imagining ourselves experiencing it calmly, in full control of our feelings and emotions... We can imagine the situation as we would like to experience it... We can see the different elements of the situation and understand the capacities we could activate to deal with it... Let's focus on the feeling of calm that comes with this image and let this sense of wellbeing spread through our body and mind..."

Take a break to absorb the exercise and finish with desophronisation.

Exercises to reduce stress

Stress is one of the most common problems facing individuals in our contemporary society, and is treated by trained sophrologists specialising in this area in individual or group sessions. During these sessions, participants learn not only how to relieve stress, but also how to prevent it, which improves the quality of their professional, family and personal lives.

More specifically, these sessions involve analysing the consequences of stress in everyday life, becoming aware of its physical and mental triggers, learning techniques to prevent and combat it, and working to develop a more positive attitude.

The following two exercises will help you to prepare to deal with a stressful situation:

• Sit with your back straight and carry out abdominal breathing and basic sophronisation. Once you have reached the sophroliminal level, carry out an exercise to displace negative elements. Next, you can carry out a visualisation of the future and imagine yourself managing a stressful moment. You will need to choose a stressful or anxiety-inducing situation to focus on, and you can prepare a *terpnos logos* text, for example:

> "We can imagine a stressful situation in the future... Let's choose a moment or an event that might be stressful for us... We are projecting ourselves fully into this moment... We are imagining ourselves experiencing it mindfully, we are imagining ourselves breathing calmly, in full control of our emotions... Let's take a step back from this moment to see it more clearly... We can think about this moment calmly, about anything that could be worrying to us and any possible solutions to these worries... Now, we can go back to the moment and imagine ourselves going through it calmly and confidently... We can let this feeling of peace wash over us..."

Finish with desophronisation. This exercise strengthens our ability to adapt and can be carried out several times a day to prepare for a stressful event.

- By visualising the colours of the rainbow, which are associated with the seven chakras (the body's energy centres according to some Eastern cultures), we can relax our body and mind before any potentially stressful situation. After a few minutes of abdominal breathing and basic sophronisation, close your eyes and visualise each colour of the rainbow in turn (red, orange, yellow, green, blue, indigo and violet). You can do this by picturing an object of each colour, taking care to choose something that you associate with feelings of pleasure or happiness. While you are thinking about each colour, associate it with a positive state, as in the following list:

- Red: physical relaxation.
- Orange: emotional relaxation.
- Yellow: mental relaxation.
- Green: inner peace.
- Blue: love and compassion.
- Indigo: alertness.
- Violet: reconnection with spirituality.

To complete the exercise, go back through the colours in reverse order, then take a break to savour your newfound sense of serenity. Finish with desophronisation.

FAQS

IS SOPHROLOGY THE SAME THING AS HYPNOSIS?

No. The philosophy on which sophrology is based is separate from hypnosis, and the patient's level of independence is not the same, as they can practise sophrology exercises alone, without the assistance of a sophrologist.

IS SOPHROLOGY THE SAME THING AS MEDITATION, YOGA OR PSYCHOANALYSIS?

No. Sophrology is a scientific method that respects the individual's personal beliefs. Unlike yoga and meditation, it is not a spiritual method. Furthermore, it does not interpret the individual's thoughts and actions in the same way as psychoanalysis, but simply promotes the positive elements of their life.

CAN I CARRY OUT SOPHROLOGY WITHOUT THE HELP OF A SOPHROLOGIST?

No. Although a course of sophrology involves some personal work that should be carried out every day, the presence of a sophrologist is vital to get the complete experience and achieve a precise objective. The sophrologist will establish a detailed, progressive programme of exercises to follow and will serve as the practitioner's "guide".

WHO CAN CARRY OUT SOPHROLOGY AND HOW DOES IT WORK?

Anyone can practise sophrology, no matter their age or level of fitness. All you need are comfortable clothes and a quiet place where you will not be disturbed for at least ten minutes per day.

HOW LONG DOES A COURSE OF SOPHROLOGY LAST?

The length of treatment depends on the problem to be treated. In general, a course of at least eight weeks, with a one-hour session each week, will enable the patient to obtain positive results in specific areas (for example, stress management, self-esteem and emotional management). However, some problems, such as panic attacks or depression, may require a longer course of treatment. Each person's situation is unique, so their programme will be tailored to them.

WHAT HAPPENS DURING A COURSE OF SOPHROLOGY?

After a preliminary interview, the sophrologist will establish the programme to follow and gradually teach the patient the necessary exercises, sometimes recording them (the recordings will then be sent to the patient by email so that they can use them to accompany the exercises they carry out at home). You will need to set aside between 10 and 20 minutes to carry out the techniques you have learnt during the sessions on your own, and these exercises must be practised regularly.

HOW CAN I BECOME A CAYCEDIAN SOPHROLOGIST?

To become a Caycedian sophrologist, you will need to follow a training course in Caycedian sophrology® and then specialise in clinical sophrology, social sophrology or sophrology for stress management and personal development. This training is held in institutions overseen by Sofrocay®, the International Caycedian Sophrology® Academy headquartered in Andorra.

We want to hear from you!
Leave a comment on your online library
and share your favourite books on social media!

FURTHER READING

BIBLIOGRAPHY

- (No date) *Académie de Sophrologie Caycédienne® Bruxelles-Luxembourg.* [Online]. [Accessed 24 July 2018]. Available from: <http://www.sophrologie.be/>

- Aliotta, C. (2014) *Manuel de sophrologie. Fondements, concepts et pratique du métier.* Paris: InterÉditions.

- Beudaert, D-P. (No date) Les théories et principes du Professeur A. Caycedo. *Sophrologie clinque.* [Online]. [Accessed 24 July 2018]. Available from: <http://www.sophrologieclinique.fr/ix-les-theories-et-principes-du-professeur-a-caycedo/>

- Chapelle, C. (2011) *La sophrologie pour les nuls.* Paris: First Éditions.

- Chéné, P-A. (2008) *Sophrologie. Fondements et méthodologie.* Vol. I. Paris: Ellébore.

- Davrou, Y. (1986) *La sophrologie facile. 30 exercices simples, relaxants et dynamisants.* Paris: Marabout.

- Etchelecou, B. (2009) *Comprendre et pratiquer la sophrologie.* Paris: InterÉditions.

- (No date) *La Chambre Syndicale de la Sophrologie*. [Online]. [Accessed 24 July 2018]. Available from: <https://www.chambre-syndicale-sophrologie.fr/>

- Payen de la Garanderie, A. (2009) *La sophrologie*. Paris: Éyrolles.

- Serrat, C. (2014) *La sophrologie c'est malin*. Paris: Leduc.s Éditions.

- (No date) *Sofrocay: Académie Internationale de Sophrologie Caycédienne*. [Online]. [Accessed 24 July 2018]. Available from: <http://www.sofrocay.com/en>

ADDITIONAL SOURCES

- Antiglio, D. (2018) *The Life-Changing Power of Sophrology: Breathe and Connect with the Calm and Happy You*. London: Yellow Kite.

- Parot, F. (2016) *Instant Serenity for Life and Work: An Introduction to Sophrology*. Ashford: Light Bubble Publishing.

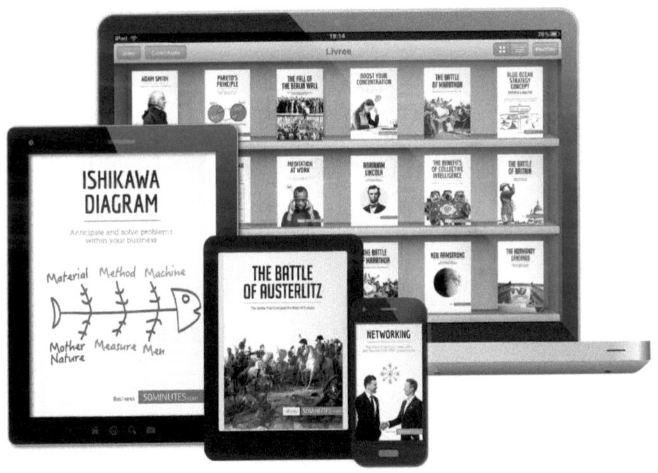

50MINUTES.com

History

Business

Coaching

Book Review

Health & Wellbeing

IMPROVE YOUR GENERAL KNOWLEDGE

IN A BLINK OF AN EYE !

www.50minutes.com

Although the editor makes every effort to verify the accuracy of the information published, 50Minutes.com accepts no responsibility for the content of this book.

© 50MINUTES.com, 2018. All rights reserved.

www.50minutes.com

Ebook EAN: 9782808011303

Paperback EAN: 9782808011310

Legal Deposit: D/2018/12603/310

Cover: © Primento

Digital conception by Primento, the digital partner of publishers.